Learning to care

EFFECTIVE GOAL SETTING

Nan Kemp
RGN, RCNT, DipN(Lond)

Nursing Consultant, Quality Assurance

Previously
Senior Nurse, Nursing Practice,
Special Projects for South West Hampshire
Health Authority

Eileen Richardson
RGN, SCM, RNT, BA(Hons)

Senior Tutor,
School of Nursing,
Salisbury Health Authority

GN00724475

© 1988 N. Kemp and E. Richardson

First published in Great Britain 1988

British Library Cataloguing Publication Data

Kemp, Nan
  Effective goal setting.
  1. Patients. Care. Planning – For nursing.
  I. Title   II. Richardson, Eileen   III. Series
  610.73

  ISBN 0 340 43009 5

Typeset in 10/11 pt Trump Medieval by
Rowland Phototypesetting Limited, Bury St Edmunds, Suffolk

Printed and bound in Great Britain
for Edward Arnold, the educational, academic
and medical publishing division of
Hodder and Stoughton Limited, 41 Bedford Square,
London WC1B 3DQ by Richard Clay Limited,
Bungay, Suffolk

LEARNING TO CARE SERIES

General Editor

JEAN HEATH, MED, BA, SRN, SCM, CERT ED

English National Board Learning Resources
Unit,
Sheffield

Titles in this series include:

Learning to Care on the Genito-urinary Ward
R BODDINGTON
Learning to Care on the Paediatric Ward
H LEWER
Learning to Care in Midwifery
J ALEXANDER
Learning to Care in the Theatre
K NIGHTINGALE
Learning to Care on the Surgical Ward
M ATTREE and J MERCHANT
Learning to Care in Community Psychiatric Nursing
M WARD and R BISHOP
Learning to Care on the Orthopaedic Ward
D JULIEN
Learning to Care on the Psychiatric Ward
M WARD
Learning to Care in the A & E Department
G JONES
Learning to Care for Elderly People
L THOMAS
Learning to Care on the Medical Ward
A MATTHEWS
Learning to Care in the Community
P TURTON and J ORR
Learning to Care on the ENT Ward
D STOKES
Learning to Care on the Gynaecology Ward
W SIMONS
Learning to Care for Mentally Handicapped People
V POUNDS

EDITOR'S FOREWORD

In most professions there is a traditional gulf between theory and its practice, and nursing is no exception. The gulf is perpetuated when theory is taught in a theoretical setting and practice is taught by the practitioner.

This inherent gulf has to be bridged by students of nursing, and publication of this series is an attempt to aid such bridge building.

It aims to help relate theory and practice in a meaningful way whilst underlining the importance of the person being cared for.

It aims to introduce students of nursing to some of the more common problems found in each new area of experience in which they will be asked to work.

It aims to de-mystify some of the technical language they will hear, putting it in context, giving it meaning and enabling understanding.

FOREWORD

The philosophy of individualised care essentially places the person who is being cared for at the centre of any plan of action and subsequent evaluation of care given. Today the theory of individualised planned care is embraced in health authorities throughout the United Kingdom; sadly, the practice in many areas is somewhat behind the theory.

One of the problem areas appears to be in the evaluating of care given. The ability to evaluate or measure effectiveness is directly related to the quality of goal setting. Adequate evaluation is essential if, as a profession, we are to accept the notion of accountability.

In *Learning to Care: Effective Goal Setting*, Nan Kemp and Eileen Richardson describe clearly and simply how goals can be set which can be measured; goals which are meaningful will also be measurable. The use of unambiguous language which anyone can understand is important. This book represents the authors' work experiences in the field, one as an educationalist and the other in clinical practice. They have both been committed over the past few years to improving the way the measurement of care is carried out. In implementing any change in an organisation the importance of good staff development must be central. The authors have been active in this field within their own organisations and offer suggestions to others with a similar task. This successful theory and practice link can only enhance the efforts to improve the service nurses offer.

1988   Jean Heath

ACKNOWLEDGEMENTS

We gratefully acknowledge the help of colleagues and friends who directly or indirectly have contributed towards the content of this book and gave constructive support in its development.

They are: Don Whittick, Gladys Law, Terri Fox, Barry Lunt, the nurses of Southampton and Salisbury Health Districts.

Gratitude is also expressed to Elaine Parker and Sarah Kemp for their patience in giving secretarial help.

NOTE

For the sake of clarity the pronoun 'she' refers to the nurse and 'he' refers to the patient. No bias is intended in the use of pronouns; we trust our readers will understand and agree with us. 'Patient' is used to represent client and resident (the person for whom we are caring).

CONTENTS

Introduction: beliefs about nursing

'Nurses are in the people business' (Whittick, 1980). They are concerned with the business of caring not just in times of illness but also when people are well. If we accept that nurses are in a business which concerns itself with people we must first establish our beliefs about man.

Man is a unique being who lives in a society where he has family and/or friends who are significant to him. The customs and cultures of that society influence his individuality as do other factors internal to him. All individuals have a variety of needs which may be classified under headings which are: physical, psychological, social and spiritual. 'A need is that which is necessary, useful or desirable to maintain homeostasis and life itself – a need becomes the motivation for behaviour' (Lewis, 1979).

If these needs are being adequately met in one's life a state of 'wellness' prevails. 'Wellness' is a balance between one's environment, internal and external, and one's emotional, social, cultural and physical processes. (Ebersole & Hess, 1981).

There are many situations in life where needs are not being met for whatever reason and this will affect the individual and cause him to behave in a variety of ways. When this happens his state of 'wellness' is reduced; the nurse may then be required to act in a variety of roles to help meet his needs. When nursing intervention becomes necessary it does not inevitably mean that the individual's independence is reduced to any great degree. We

1

believe that the individual should be consulted and involved in the decisions which are made about his care and participate meaningfully in those aspects of his care which are appropriate. The patient's family and friends may also be involved in the assessment of his needs and the plan for his care, so that realistic decisions are taken which are based both on the nurse's knowledge and experience and on the patient and his family's information. In this way the patient is more likely to reach a set goal of care because he and his family know what is expected of him.

In nursing there are those who feel that models or conceptual frameworks are useful ways of organising one's thinking. They may certainly help to create a more informed basis for using the nursing process and therefore we should choose a model which is appropriate for the person whose care we are planning.

As our philosophy of nursing is embedded in the concept that man is an individual, it is for this reason that we feel that in the organisation of care an individualised approach must be used. We see in the nursing process such an approach. As it is a systematic way of thinking about and implementing nursing care it allows for logical planning. It also allows for measurement of the effectiveness of care which is so important in these days when, as the UKCC *Code of Professional Conduct* reminds us, 'each registered nurse, midwife and health visitor is accountable for his or her practice. . . .' We are expected to control our performance to ensure that the care we provide is 'the best possible within the available resources'. (DHSS HC (84) 13).

The following steps in this process are now familiar to most nurses:

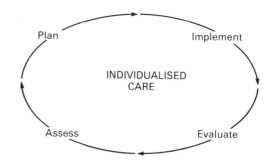

Framework for the nursing process. (Based on Heath & Law, 1982)

At the assessment interview, and in the planning phase we are concerned to identify the problems and needs of the individual in our care. When this has been done we need to set against each problem the goal or anticipated outcome which our care is expected to achieve. This is often an area of weakness in the planning cycle. If goals are not clearly set we may have difficulty in correctly evaluating the patient's progress and our practice.

It is for this reason that we have set ourselves the task of preparing a book which we hope will be of practical use to nurses and one which will in the end improve their ability to evaluate the care they give.

COMMUNI-CATION

If we believe that the patient has responsibility for his own health state, then he should, whenever possible, be involved in decision-making regarding his care, for it is more likely that the patient will make the most use of a nursing contribution to this care if he has been involved in seeing how his contribution was arrived at. He will have a much greater sense of contributing to his own care by 'doing with' rather than 'being done to'. If we are to effectively use goals in the evaluation of care then we must be sure that everyone, but in particular the patient, knows and understands the goals. Herein lie a great many difficulties that nurses face with care planning, because they traditionally see and write the care plan in terms of themselves rather than in those of the patient.

The ability to accurately communicate goals is important not just between the nurse and the patient but also between the nurse and his family. Families are usually part of the patient's support system, therefore their contribution should be taken into account. Members of a family can only participate appropriately in the patient's care if they are involved in the decision making.

Experience shows that in psychiatry, for example, the patient's problems are sometimes seen to be rooted within the family, so that involving them from the beginning in the patient's plan is not just a bonus but a necessity.

Communication with others

It is imperative for the continuation of good care that accurate information is available not just for the nurse who designed the care plan, but for all who share and are concerned with care in her absence. It may be that in the case of changing shifts or days off, another trained nurse takes over the care. She may have her own ideas about how care should be given, but in the interest of the patient it is important that continuity is maintained based on accurately set goals. Learner nurses may have

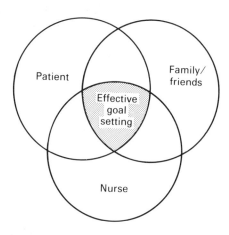

Complete communication is necessary for effective goal setting

aspects of planning care delegated to them, however they should not have the responsibility of making the final decision about care, although they do need to learn how care may be planned. In the planning cycle the goal setting element is often seen to be the most difficult.

Bank and Agency nurses are often employed in our hospitals. It is important that they too are educated to recognise the importance of accurate goal setting and can appreciate the rationale behind the planning of care. There is no doubt that in the circumstances described above, the written plan, with its goals clearly stated, is necessary to maintain the patient's and the nurse's confidence.

We know that planned transfers are necessary at times, for example, from Intensive to Continuing care or from Assessment to Rehabilitation wards, therefore it is important to ensure that the care plan is transferred with the patient so that nurses on the different areas can see what goals have been set and how far they have been met at the time of transfer. The patient is going to feel there is genuine concern for him where he sees that the plan of care continues to receive attention and that it reflects his current condition and concerns.

Disciplines other than nursing are also involved in care, for example physiotherapists and occupational therapists also identify problems and needs of patients and plan appropriate care to meet prescribed goals.

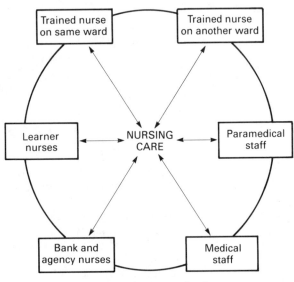

Communicating with others

To ensure that the patient has the maximum benefit from any goal setting exercise, it is important that each member of the care team should know of each other's plan for care and ideally be working towards achieving the patient's goals for the maximum benefit of the patient. The need to improve communication, and therefore congruence, in goal setting is illustrated clearly by Lunt and Neale (1985) in their work on goal setting in the care of the terminally ill patient. This work involved a study of goal setting in two hospices and one district general hospital setting. In these three settings they compared goals and outcomes of goals set by nurses and by doctors, in the expectation that the better the communication between staff, the more congruent would be the views of the team's aims.

Their findings showed differences between goals set by doctors and those set by nurses in the district general hospital but not in the hospices, leading to different expectations of outcomes. They conclude that there is a 'need for better communication between doctors and nurses in hospital to co-ordinate care plans'.

The more precise and realistic the goal setting by the nurse, the easier it will be for health care colleagues to work alongside her, helping the patient to reach these goals by using their special skills; the easier, too, these same colleagues may find it to follow the reasoning behind the nursing interventions. Clearly, time spent in the preparations for goal setting by detailed assessment and problem identification pays dividends, improving the accuracy of goal setting and communication with others in the caring team.

2 The process of goal setting

WHAT IS
A GOAL?

goal *n.* **1.** point marking end of race; object of effort or ambition; destination. **2.** pair of posts between which ball is to be driven in football . . .
The Concise Oxford Dictionary, 1982

Whilst we have chosen to use the word *goal*, many other nurses use *objective, desired outcome, expected outcome* and *target*. All these words can be said to have the same meaning when referring to nursing care. Little and Carnevali (1976) refer to the words patients may use when discussing the goals of care; some of these are *hopes, aims, wants, wishes, purposes* and *ambitions*. This is a useful list to remember when discussing goals of care with the patient.

Some definitions that may be of use are as follows:

A goal is a statement of a desired, achievable outcome to be attained within a predicted period of time, given the presenting situation and resources. (Little & Carnevali, 1976)

A goal means what a person will be doing as a result of care and/or treatment which is different and better than at present. (Lunt, 1986)

A goal statement should contain:

an *observation* of something that the patient expresses or *behaviour* that he will be able to do;

a *measurement* and *time constraint* that enables an evaluation of the patient's progress and care to be carried out;

and it should be *achievable* and *appropriate* for the patient and the resources available.

As previously indicated, formulating and writing goals appears to give many people difficulty, for too often, as Lunt (1978) points out, 'Goals are implicit or intuitive, rather than explicit, which can leave others in the dark, including the patient'. Often goals are written as aims, or what Mager (1975) calls 'Fuzzies'. We have all seen such examples: 'to be mobilised', 'wound to heal', 'to be rehydrated', 'to have quality of life'. There is nothing wrong in principle with these statements; they often reflect the philosophy of the people writing them. However, they are almost impossible to measure and evaluate effectively.

HOW TO SET GOALS

Goals contain a statement about some activity the patient will carry out or that will occur as a result of care or therapy. It therefore follows that before writing the goal statement the nurse should discuss with the patient his problems and needs. She should ask, when appropriate to do so, what sort of change he would like to see as a result of the care he is going to receive. Together they will discuss how the goal is to be achieved and the kind of nursing action and treatment that will take place to aid the achievement of the goal. Whilst the nurse, through her knowledge, experience and analysis of the assessment data can guide the goal setting, it is only after discussion with the patient or significant others that his resources can be identified to enable him to reach the goal. 'Resources' in this context means the help he is likely to give or obtain from others, such as family, friends or the support services, for without such help it is unlikely that some goals will be achieved.

However, not all patients can or wish to be involved in identifying their problems or needs, let alone the setting of goals. Where the patient lacks the ability to be involved and has no-one to speak for him, the nurse takes on this role. To involve the patient who is disinterested and/or does not have the will to be involved is also difficult.

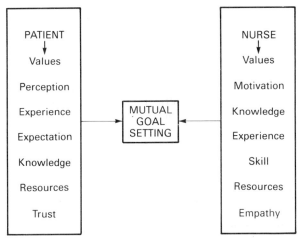

Factors influencing mutual goal setting

In most situations the nurse's relationship with the patient and her skill may enable her to overcome some of the difficulties. But whatever the circumstances, the nurse still has to capitalise on any strengths the patient may have or has had.

One of the advantages of goal setting is that

it can act as a stimulus for the patient – something that gives him a sense of purpose, something to work for. For example: Mr John Brown, a patient with bone metastasis, was at home receiving terminal care. He was being cared for by his wife, Anne, and the district nurse. He had become withdrawn and was apparently not interested in anything and said as much. He just wanted 'to get it over with'. Anne and the nurse discussed how they could help him. Anne said that he had been a keen gardener until recently. It was suggested to John that he plan a flower garden with Anne and supervise her carrying out the work. This they did together. He sat in a chair whilst she dug the garden and planted the seeds. There is no doubt that these activities, which were achieved through a series of goal steps, enabled the patient to reach the goal, 'Planned and supervised the planting of a flower garden by 21 March, 1988'.

This example shows how, by discussing a problem and identifying a patient's strengths (in this case his love for his wife and his past interest), it was possible to motivate the patient and give him and his wife something to work for, which obviously helped them both. It also enabled the patient, his wife and the nurse to plan other goals.

Writing a goal statement (Based on Mager, 1975)

A goal may contain the following:

1   *Performance* – the actual behaviour, communication or clinical features demonstrated by the patient, e.g. *walks*; *recognises*; *writes*; *reports*; *decreasing weight*.

2   *Condition* – the environment or help required from a person and or resources, e.g.

with the aid of the Zimmer Frame; *supported by daughter*; *in the hall.*

3 *Criteria* – the measurement – how well, how long, how far, how often, how much, e.g. walks with the Zimmer Frame *from the hall to the door twice a day.* Loss of weight – *1 kg in one week.*

4 *Target* – the predicted time by which the goal will be achieved and thus evaluated.

5 *Review* – a checking time may be necessary for some long term goals, when an evaluation statement should also be written.

Goals may be classified according to three types of time constraint; *immediate, short term* and *long term.*

Immediate

An immediate goal would be necessary for such situations as: preoperative and postoperative care, diabetic coma, convulsion, etc. May be written in minutes/hours, according to the patient's condition, for example:

Problem: potential shock, following operation.

Goals in this case could include: warm, dry skin; stable blood pressure 130/80 mmHg −140.90 mmHg; pulse rate 60–90 beats per minute, regular and strong; resting quietly; no bright red, blood-saturated dressing. Review every 15 minutes.

Short term

A short term goal is used for any situation where a resolution of the problem can more or less be predicted, for example:

Problem: a newly diagnosed diabetic 1.2.88. Lacks the skill to test urine.

Goal: demonstrate correct method of testing urine using clinitest kit, recording and reporting results accurately by 3.2.88.

Long term

The length of time may be in weeks or even months for psychological, social, spiritual and chronic physical problems, for example: breakdown in relationships, abnormal grief reaction, alcohol dependence, loneliness, bizzare behaviour, stroke, loss of vision and varicose ulcers.

When setting goals for the long term problem, it is advisable to break them down into manageable parts. These are usually referred to as goal steps or sub goals and can be achieved in a shorter space of time than the long term goal.

GOAL STEPS

From the patient's point of view he is much more likely to be interested in working towards something he can see is achievable in a short space of time, than the long term goal which could be reached some time in the future. In this way too the patient will be working at a pace in keeping with his predicted progress.

As one goal step is achieved the nurse and, if possible, the patient will together evaluate progress so far and discuss the feasibility of moving on to the next step. Goal steps therefore not only help to motivate the patient, but ensure that evaluation is systematically carried out at predetermined intervals. This is a more effective procedure than waiting for the achievement of the long term goal or for something unexpected to happen.

How many goal steps do you write? There are no hard or fast rules – it depends on the patient, his condition and the resources available, together with the nurse's skill and experience in dealing with the particular problem. Goal steps for some problems can more or less be predicted, as in the example given on page 12. However, for the more protracted problem, it can at times be difficult to predict the time span for the achievement of the long term goal or even the goal steps required. Therefore it is sensible to write only one or two goal steps to be achieved in a specific time. As progress is evaluated and goals are achieved, further goal steps may be written. Thus, sub goals or goal steps may be written as illustrated in the following example.

EXAMPLE

Mr Brian Smith is a 72-year-old married man. He lives with his wife who is devoted to him. A married daughter lives close by. Six months ago Mr Smith suffered a stroke which left him with a right-sided hemiplegia. He made a good recovery and was discharged from hospital four months ago. His wife says he has recently become reluctant to use his walking aid following a slight fall.

The care plan on page 16 shows the various goal steps used for Mr Smith.

If we remember to involve the patient and his family in problem identification in the setting of goal steps, the outcome is more likely to be successful.

Date	Problem	Goals
1.2.88	Reluctant to walk using walking aid following slight fall. (Has right-sided hemiplegia.)	Walks from armchair to sitting room door twice each day on his own using a Zimmer Frame. Review 13.2.88.
		Walks from armchair to front door twice each day using Zimmer Frame. Review 20.2.88.
		States he is confident to walk to shop with his wife by 26.2.88.
		Walks to shop using Zimmer Frame and accompanied by his wife Tuesday and Friday. Review 5.3.88.
		Walks to daughter's house for tea and returns without difficulty. Review 12.3.88.
		Resumes routine of walking to shop and visiting daughter – using walking aid. By 1.4.88.

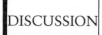

DISCUSSION

Some nurses may choose to use the patient's name when writing goals. However, if the care plan is centred on the patient, is this necessary? Nevertheless at times the person giving help will need to be named, for example: Accepts daughter's help to get in and out of bath. 1.4.88.

Performance

All goals *must* have a *performance*. This can be the observed 'patient behaviour' or activity, i.e. what he reports or says, what he does. It may also be a clinical manifestation which is not necessarily under the control of the patient, such as normal temperature, weight loss, decreasing decubitus ulcer. A goal statement carries more impact if it starts with a verb: states, demonstrates, listens, smiles, writes, reduces, contrasts, selects, washes. It is not always necessary to write a condition for a goal, for example:

Problem: 1.4.88 Dry mouth.
Goal: Clean moist buccal mucosa by 2.4.88.

Criterion

A goal statement *must* have a *criterion*, for this is the indicator for evaluating how effective the care of the patient has been and how he has responded to that care. It is also worth noting that the writing of measurable goals should enable nurses to be more effective when they set and measure nursing standards.

Target date

This is the predicted time when the goal will be achieved and an evaluation made and written. It will be in part influenced by the nurse's knowledge and experience and the patient's condition, motivation and resources. It must be realistic, meaning the patient should be able to achieve the goal by the stated time. Some target dates are not easy to predict, as we said earlier, particularly with long term goals; however if they are broken down into manageable parts (goal steps) this problem can be overcome.

Review date

It may on occasion be necessary to set a review date – a time that progress is checked and a statement written. To set a date, be this target or review, is essential, for this is a specific and disciplined way of ensuring care is evaluated.

of problems and goals

Here are some further examples of problems and goals which may be of help to you. However, it should be remembered that goals are individual to patients because of their particular needs and resources. It does not follow that the type of problem stated here will necessarily have the goals we have set in each case.

Date	Problem	Goals
1.3.88	Potential bleeding due to predicted long term administration of warfarin tablets.	Lists accurately the side effects and action to be taken on 3.3.88. States he can cope if side effects occur. By 3.3.88.
1.3.88	Potential hypoglycaemic attacks due to instability of blood glucose level (newly diagnosed diabetic).	Experiences hypoglycaemic attack under controlled conditions. By 2.3.88. Lists correctly actions to prevent and deal with hypoglycaemic attack. By 3.3.88. States he is confident to deal with hypoglycaemia after discharge from hospital. By 5.3.88.
1.3.88	Passing hard, dry stools twice weekly.	Regains normal bowel action and pattern of once daily. By 7.3.88.
1.3.88	Outbursts of verbal and physical aggression at least twice every hour.	Time between outbursts extended to two hours. Review daily. Target date 5.3.88.

Date	Problem	Goals
1.3.88	Disorientated with regard to time.	Accurately reports to Primary Nurse each morning the date, time and place. Review daily.
1.3.88	Overweight by 12.5 kg (awaiting cardiac surgery).	Reduce weight by 3 kg first week – 7.3.88. Reduce weight thereafter by 1.5 kg weekly. Review weekly. Achieves target weight of 85 kg. By 5.4.88.

3 Evaluation procedure

Evaluation is a part of the cycle of the nursing process when we judge the effectiveness or otherwise of nursing action towards goal achievements. Evaluation means 'to determine the value of something' (Chambers, 1980). It is at times a complex process calling for an analysis of information that we perceive by our senses, and its interpretation is based on experience, knowledge and our value system.

Fortunately, the goal setting approach to care used today, with its measurable criteria, should make evaluation easier than in the past. When taking a broad perspective of evaluation it is a help to keep in mind Donabedian's (1969), Triad of Structure, Process and Outcome, which was developed to aid the evaluation of medical care, illustrated on page 22.

Structure is concerned with the evaluation of the conditions under which care and service are provided, e.g. the buildings, equipment, staff, time available and management style.

Process is when the evaluator looks at what the health carer does to and for the patient, and how.

Outcome is the result of the care on the patient.

The triad is a useful framework to keep in mind when analysing progress towards

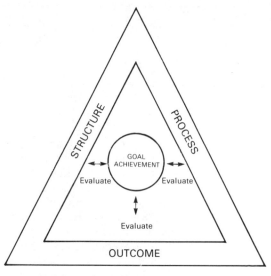

Framework for evaluating goal setting achievement. (Based on Donabedian, 1969)

the goal achievement itself, for we can ask ourselves:
a) were the resources adequate? (structure);
b) how did the nurse carry out the care? (process); and
c) what effect did it have on the patient? (outcome).

Evaluation is often thought of as the last stage in the nursing process. This is not always so, for we are evaluating the effectiveness of care from the time care begins. For example, we judge how well a patient responds when he gets out of bed for the first time after an operation, or how well a wound is healing and how competent a new mother is in bathing her baby. This is known as *formative* evaluation, which is sometimes written on a review date. *Summative* evaluation is made when the goal, or the sum of the goals, is achieved or care is discontinued. This is when the total plan of care should be evaluated, thus evaluation statements can be seen as a record of the consequences of care.

All evaluation statements should be written, dated and signed by the person making the evaluation. Ideally this should be the nurse who has set the goals with the patient and/or has had the responsibility for his care, for she should have the most knowledge about the patient. Indeed, there may be occasions when the patient will write down his own evaluation. His responses will enable a more effective and realistic evaluation to be carried out. Photographs and drawings may sometimes be used as a record of progress and thus of evaluation.

THE EVALU-ATION PROCEDURE

1 Check goal statement on review or target date.
2 Collect information – Table 3.1 might be useful as a source of reference.
3 Consult patient and, if necessary, significant others.
4 Make a judgement.
5 Evaluation will include one of the following:
   a) goal achieved
   b) goal no longer relevant
   c) goal not yet achieved.

Comment

If the result is 'goal achieved' it is wise to check if the goal was pertinent to the problem and if the problem has been resolved or modified to such an extent that no further progress is required or possible.

'Goal no longer relevant' may mean that the patient's condition has changed to such an extent that he no longer can or even needs to reach the goal because the problem has changed or ceased to exist.

'Goal not yet achieved' may mean that the time for evaluation was unrealistic or that the patient's condition has changed, making the resolution of the problem slower than anticipated. When analysing the reason for this it would be useful to check if the problem is still the same, or if the nursing action was correct.

CHECKLIST

1 *Check problem definition*
—Does the patient still have the problem?
—Is the problem clearly stated with descriptions that enable a measurement to take place when necessary, and that there is no area for misinterpretation, as this could lead to inappropriate goal setting? For example:
    Poor mobility
    Anxious
    Spits at people
    Large varicose ulcer
—Does the patient acknowledge or understand his problem?
—Has the patient been told about his problem?

Table 3.1 Aids to evaluation

Records	Observation	Communications	Measurement
Reports	Look	Talking	Measuring utensils for fluids
Care plans	Touch	Listening	
Notes	Listen	Touching	Watch
Flow charts	Smell	Observing	Thermometer
Graphs		Non-verbal clues	Sphygmomanometer
Scales			Scales
Photographs			Ruler
Drawings			Chemical analysis
			Graphs
			Camera

2   *Analysis of prescribed nursing action as written in the care plan*

Ask yourself the following questions:

—Are the instructions clearly stated?

—Are the instructions realistic for the patient and the resources available?

—Are the instructions still applicable for this particular problem?

—Have any changes in the care been noted and at the correct time?

—Are the instructions being followed; if not, why not? It is wise to check previous evaluation statements and progress notes, also check with colleagues if there is any doubt whether written instructions are being followed.

—Are all the people referred to in the instructions involved; if not, why not?

—Is the equipment available to enable care to be carried out?

—Are the actions based on outmoded practices and therefore inappropriate and hindering goal achievement?

—Does the patient know what is expected of him? If he does not, this too may hinder goal achievement.

It is sensible when analysing prescribed nursing actions to check if the frequency of goal review and resultant changes in any prescription have been noted in the action column.

If, finally, you have checked the goal problem and action and everything seems correct, please 'relook' at the goal statement for there is probably a need to reset the time limits.

In Module 5 of *Systematic Approach to Nursing Care* (Open University, 1984) it is pointed out that goals that remain static can be a positive sign when applied to potential problems, for it is a sign of success if the situation does not change. This can mean that the patient's condition is improving, and/or that the preventative and checking measures are being effective in preventing the occurrence of the potential problem.

How to measure

It has been noted earlier that all goal statements must have criteria. There are times when a physical measurement can be used, which makes evaluation of the effectiveness of care much easier and more precise. In order to effect this measurement different 'tools' may be used. Sometimes these tools may be instruments designed specifically for the purpose:

> Jugs and graduated measuring utensils for fluid.
> Watch for timing pulse and respiration.
> Thermometer to measure temperature.
> Sphygmomanometer to measure blood pressure.
> Scales to measure weight.
> Tape measure/ruler to measures distance.
> Reagent strip for chemical analysis.
> Charts and graphs to measure frequency and demonstrate clinical observations.
> Camera for photographs of posture, wounds, etc.

Measuring cards using sterile material to assess changes in the size of pressure sores may also be designed.

One method of dealing with a record of changing frequencies, for example, when measuring bowel actions, wound drainage, vomiting, convulsions etc., might be to represent them by use of a bar chart or histogram. For example, if a goal was related to the reduction in the number of convulsions a patient was having, progress towards the goal might be recorded on a chart such as follows.

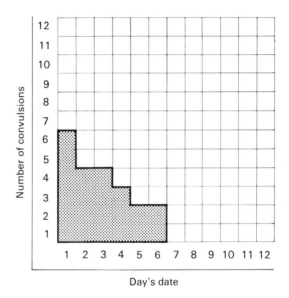

Day's date

Chart to measure frequency of convulsions

The nurse would be able to fill in one section of the chart when each convulsion was observed giving a total at the end of the 24 hours or whenever was appropriate.

Graphic illustration is also useful in indicating recorded changes in temperature, blood pressure, pattern of incontinence, sleep patterns. In this case a linear representation is used.

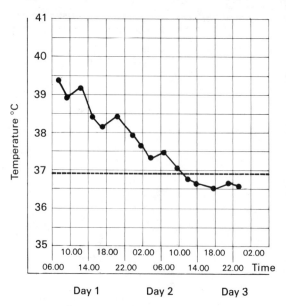

Graph to demonstrate clinical observations

Where subjective information is in the goal's statement, as when the patient reports a feeling, a thought and reacts to something, it is sometimes possible also to use a 'tool' which makes evaluation easier; scales which monitor, for example, *pain*, *anxiety* and *mood*.

Points on these scales are agreed by discussion with the patient. They are then used to indicate the effectiveness of the care and in so doing the progress towards the stated goal. It is a wise investment to search for such tools that have been validated by use and in research, for example the Glasgow Coma Scale as shown in McFarlane & Castledene (1982).

PAIN SCALE

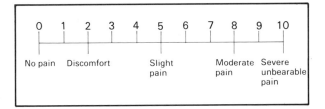

ANXIETY SCALE

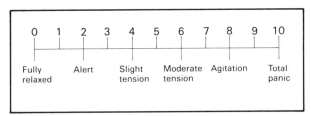

Actual measurements will be set in agreement with the patient and using his words

Writing the evaluation statement

As previously indicated, the evaluation statement will refer to the patient's actual status in relation to the goal on the target or review date.

It is also evident that a statement may need to be made outside the planned dates if anything unusual happens to the patient. A written statement will be noted in the evaluation column on the care plan, progress notes or medical notes, whichever is the choice of the organisation. The problem definition, the goal statement and the nursing prescription (action column) should be reviewed and changed if necessary.

What to write

If the goal has been achieved the statement can read – 'goal achieved'. However, a short statement saying *what* the goal achieved gives a clearer picture of the result of care, for example:

Drank 3 litres of fluid in 24 hours
or   Gained 4 kg in weight

Remember to date and sign the evaluation statement.

If the goal has not been achieved but remains relevant, perhaps because progress is slower than anticipated, it is necessary to write a short evaluation statement and set a new review or target date. At times, particularly with goal steps, a statement referring to the criteria within the goal is all that is necessary, such as:

Ulcer now 5 cm by 2.5 cm
or   Reduction in weight 1 kg

On occasions it may be necessary to write a more detailed statement about the patient's response, for example, the evaluation statement for the patient mentioned on page 12 read:

Sat in chair without discomfort whilst Anne prepared the seed bed – joking about her crooked rows 'like a dog's hind leg'.

When you consider what the patient's problem was you can see that he became less withdrawn and responded to his surroundings.

Evaluation statements may at times also mention such things as changes in care, but not in any detail, as this will go in the nursing prescription (action) column.

Many nurses cross through the problem, goal and the nursing prescription when the goal is achieved or the problem ceases to exist. However, the nursing record is classified as a primary document and 'it will form a permanent part of the patient's case folder together with other documents'. Amongst other things it is 'a source of information about the patient. It is an aid to teaching and research. It can be used for legal purposes'. (King's Fund Project, No. 21, 1979). The primary document is stored for many years after the last date of entry. It therefore follows that the information on the nursing record should be available, accurate and legible. Information should not be erased; if it is crossed through, it should be a thin ink line, enabling the words underneath to be seen. The procedure to be followed should be dictated by District, Hospital or Unit policy.

Accountability

Whereas all levels of nurses may be involved in carrying out care and thus provide information that will enable evaluation to take place, it is the trained nurse together with the learner nurse, the patient, and significant others who should make the final judgement about the success or otherwise towards goal achievement. The trained nurse will be the person to write the evaluation statement although the learner nurse may do this if it is checked by a trained nurse.

Conclusion

The foregoing discussion leads us to identify the features and advantages of effective goal setting as follows:

1   Encourages discussion between the patient

and the nurse, enabling them to set goals and to identify the resources available.

2   Increases the patient's knowledge of his care.

3   Involves and motivates the patient and/or the nurse by describing the performance or observation to be made.

4   Enables the nurse and patient to organise their activities to reach the goal.

5   Involves the patient in the evaluation of care.

6   Communicates the intention of the care process to all those involved in that care, by writing goal statements that are explicit and measurable.

7   Enables an evaluation of the effectiveness of the patient's progress and nursing care to be carried out in a systematic manner.

8   Increases nursing knowledge and practice which should lead to the setting of standards and the use of criteria.

4 Summary exercises

We have included a few situations where problems have been identified so that you can test whether your goal setting skills have improved. However, before you attempt the exercises, consider the background information and the problem definition, then write a goal for each problem, including goal steps if you think it necessary. An example of a blank care plan form, including the nursing action and evaluation columns, is given at the end of this chapter for you to fill in if you would find it helpful. Please turn to page 37 when you have completed the exercises.

1 John is 42 years old and is a long-stay patient in a psychiatric hospital. He has great difficulty in managing his own life and is not able to cope with living with others in a community. In particular he cannot manage his money, so that when he needs cigarettes or other items he simply steals from other patients.

   Problem: John takes items he needs from other patients when he has spent his own money.
   Goal:

2 Margaret Smith is 20 years old and a student at the local college. She is suffering from an acute attack of ulcerative colitis, which she finds very disturbing, both emotionally and physically, as she sleeps badly, being concerned that she may soil the bed linen. Three particular problems have been identified:

a) *Problem*: Persistent copious diarrhoea.
   Goal:
b) *Problem*: Anxiety about possible faecal incontinence.
   Goal:
c) *Problem*: Awake for 10–15 minutes every two hours in the night.
   Goal:

3 Betty Wilson is 50 years old and has been having haematemesis from bleeding oesophageal varices. This has now settled, but she continues to be cared for in the medical ward until her general condition improves. There is a risk of further haemorrhage.

   Problem: Potential bleeding from oesophageal varices.
   Goal:

4 Peter Brown is 70 years old; his wife died one month ago after a long illness. Mr Brown has now been admitted with a cerebral vascular accident, which has left him with a right hemiparesis. He is depressed and withdrawn, although able to speak normally. He used to attend church regularly up until his wife's illness but his daughter says he blames God for her death.

   a) *Problem*: Withdrawn and sad due to the death of his wife.
      Goal:
   b) *Problem*: Loss of faith 'in church and God'.
      Goal:

5 Beryl is 19 years old. She is resident in a Mental Handicap Hostel where she has lived for five years. Both her parents are dead.

Beryl's strengths include: She knows and likes all members of the staff. Beryl enjoys watching the television, washing the dishes and having baths. She feeds herself without difficulty and dresses herself, but slowly. She is continent.

Beryl's difficulties include: Lack of concentration. Very little speech. She is frightened of going outside the house. Her sleep pattern is variable – sometimes she walks around in the night crying to herself. She dislikes the other female residents and if they sit close to her she pulls their hair violently.

Problem: Pulls other female residents' hair if they sit too close.
Goal:

6 John is ten years of age and is nervous in the presence of strangers. He has been in hospital for four days having sustained a fractured femur. His parents, brother aged twelve and sister aged six visit regularly and are affectionate towards him. He is making a good recovery from his surgery, however, he wets the bed at night. (His mother had warned the nurse that he had enuresis.) He is embarrassed by this, particularly as he is in a ward of children of similar ages.

Problem: Wets the bed at night.
Goal:

7 Diana is 23 years of age, and her baby is three days old. Diana is unmarried with no permanent male partner. She is a secretary by profession and lives alone in a modern rented flat in a pleasant environment. She is estranged from her parents who disapprove of her keeping the baby. She plans to employ a baby minder whilst she is

at work – but she feels guilty about this. She also admits to being frightened that she won't care for the baby properly. She appears unduly anxious when she holds the baby, although she is very loving towards the child.

Problem: 'Frightened' about coping with the baby at home on her own.
Goal:

8   Charles is a 43-year-old man with tetra-plegia who lives at home with his wife and daughter. They are given support by the district nurse who normally visits twice a week. Charles has redness of the skin on his sacral area.

Problem: Redness of the skin on sacral area.

Shape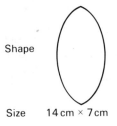

Size   14 cm × 7 cm

Goal:

Now that you have attempted the exercises check that you have considered the following points in each case:

1 Consider whether the problem was clearly understood.

2 Does your goal statement contain:
   a) performance – the behaviour or clinical feature and or communication expressed by the patient?
   b) a condition – the environment or the resources such as help from a relative?
   c) a criterion – measurement?
   d) a target or review date?
   All goal statements must contain a, c and d.

3 Did you consider whether your goal required 'goal steps' if it was long term?

4 Do you feel your goal statement is realistic in relation to the background information you were given?

5 Have you written the goal in language that everyone will clearly understand – including the patient?

CARE PLAN

Date	Problem	Goals	Nursing action	Evaluation/date

	CARE PLAN				
Date	Problem	Goals	Nursing action	Evaluation/date

5 A workshop on goal setting

This is based on the experience of the authors. It is put forward as a workable framework which has been tried but which others might like to adapt or modify to suit their own setting and participants.

AIM OF THE WORKSHOP

To improve the goal setting skills of all nurses involved in care planning.

Objectives for the participants of the workshop

At the end of the workshop the participants will be able to:

1 Define goal/objective/outcome.
2 Identify a client's problems/needs that will be used in the goal setting exercise.
3 List the factors which must be considered in goal setting.
4 Write goals for three of the problems which have been defined.
5 Discuss the need to involve all significant others in goal setting for the client.
6 Write a long and a short-term goal for two particular problems.
7 Discuss the need to include a time element in goal setting.
8 Describe the relationship between goal setting and the evaluation of care.

Pre-reading

Two weeks prior to the workshop, participants will be sent a reading list, for example *Goal Analysis* by Robert Mager (1984).

Duration and structure of the workshop

The workshop will be of one day's duration, approximately 9.30 a.m.–4.30 p.m.

Participants should be instructed beforehand to bring with them information about patients which will enable a variety of problems to be identified, against which goals can be set. It would be particularly helpful for the participants to bring those that they have previously had difficulty with for consideration by the group.

The day consists of short presentations by the group leader, followed by general discussions interspersed with individual and group activities. It is essential that the students actually do work at writing goals to get the greatest benefit from the workshop.

Suggested outline for the day

9.15 a.m.   *Introduction by leader*
Outlining the structure of the day and the objective of the workshop.

9.30 a.m.   *Group discussion*
Identifying difficulties members have had with goal setting in the past.

10.00 a.m.   COFFEE

10.30 a.m.   *Short presentation by group leader*
Goal setting in the context of care planning.

11.00 a.m.	*Individual exercises* Re-identifying problems/needs, using information brought to the workshop, followed by group discussion.
11.30 a.m.	*Short presentation by leader* Goals – definitions, points to be considered in goal setting.
12 noon	*Individual exercises* Setting goals against previously identified problems/needs, followed by discussion involving consideration of goals written by the members of the group.
1.00 p.m.	LUNCH
2.00 p.m.	*Group work* Three or four subgroups given situations with clients by group leader for discussion within the group, leading to problem identification, goal setting.
3.00 p.m.	*Presentation of results of group exercise*, with general discussion.
3.30 p.m.	TEA
3.45 p.m.	*Summing up* by group leader.
4.00 p.m.	*Evaluation* of the day.

References

CHAMBERS TWENTIETH CENTURY DICTIONARY. 1980. Ed. A. M. Mac-Donald. Edinburgh: W. R. Chambers Ltd.

CONCISE OXFORD DICTIONARY, THE. 1982. Eds. H. W. & F. G. Fowler.

DHSS HEALTH CIRCULAR (84) 13 *Health Service Management.* Implementation of the NHS Management Inquiry Report. June 1984.

DONABEDIAN, A. 1969. Some issues in evaluating the quality of nursing care. *American Journal of Public Health.* **59**. 1833–36.

EBERSOLE, P. & HESS, P. 1981. *Towards Healthy Ageing.* London: C. V. Mosby Co.

HEATH, J. & LAW, G. M. 1982. *Nursing Process – What is it?* Sheffield: NHS Learning Resources Unit, 7.

KING'S FUND PROJECT PAPER – A handbook for nurse to nurse report. 1979. No. 21. March. London: King's Fund Centre.

LEWIS, L. W. 1979. *Fundamentals of Nursing.* Philadelphia: J. B. Lippincott Co.

LITTLE, D. E. & CARNEVALI, D. L. 1976. *Nursing Care Planning.* 2nd Ed. Philadelphia: J. B. Lippincott Co.

LUNT, B. J. 1978. *The Goal Setting Approach in Continuing Care.* Paper presented at Annual Therapeutic Conference, St Christopher's Hospice, Sydenham. 17 November. 3.

LUNT, B. J. & NEALE, C. 1985. A comparison of hospice and hospital care goals set by staff. *Palliative Medicine* Vol. 1, No. 2. 1987.

LUNT, B. J. 1986. Terminal care: goal setting – hospice philosophy in practice. *Current Issues in Clinical Psychology.* Vol. 3. Ed. E. Karas. Plenum, 1987.

MCFARLANE, Baroness of Llandaff & CASTLEDENE, G. 1982. *A Guide to the Practice of Nursing Using the Nursing Process.* London: C. V. Mosby Co.

MAGER, R. F. 1975. *Preparing Instructional Objectives.* 2nd Ed. Belmont, California: Fearon Pitman Publishers.

MAGER, R. F. 1984. *Goal Analysis.* Belmont, California: Fearon Pitman Publishers.

OPEN UNIVERSITY. 1984. *Systematic Approach to Nursing Care – An Introduction.* Open University Learning/Teaching Package. Module 5. Open University Press.

UKCC. 1984. *Code of Professional Conduct.* 2nd Ed. London.

WHITTICK, D. 1980. *Nurse Education and Rheumatology.* Paper presented at the Rheumatology Conference, Harrogate. December.

Bibliography

BARNETT, D. 1985. Making your plans work. *Nursing Times*, **81**/9 January, 24–27.

BERGMAN, R. 1982. Evaluation of nursing care: Could it make a difference? *International Journal of Nursing Studies*, **19**, 2, 53–60. ·

DAVIS, A. D. N. & CRISP, A. G. 1980. Setting performance goals in geriatric nursing. *Journal of Advanced Nursing*, **5**. 381–8.

DE LA CUESTA, C. 1983. The Nursing Process: From development to implementation. *Journal of Advanced Nursing*, **8**, 865–71.

FLEMING, I. & TOSH, M. 1985. Monitoring the nursing process: going for goals. *Nursing Mirror*, 15 May, **160**(20), 42–5.

HEATH, J., LAW, G. & CROSS, I. 1983. *Nursing Process – What is it!* (Adapted for Psychiatric Nursing.) Sheffield: ENB Learning Resources Unit.

HEATH, J., GREEN, J., LAW, G. & FRAZER, P. 1985. *Nursing Process – What is it!* (Adapted for Mental Handicap Nursing.) Sheffield: ENB Learning Resources Unit.

HEATH, J., LAW, G. M. & KEMP, N. 1986. *Introducing Change – Nursing Process in Practice.* Sheffield: ENB Learning Resources Unit.

HUNT, J. M. & MARKS-MARAN, D. J. 1980. *Nursing Care Plans: the Nursing Process at Work.* London: HM & M Publishers.

KEMP, N. 1984. *Quality Assurance and the Nursing Process.* Study Tour Report. Florence Nightingale/Smith & Nephew Scholarship. London: Florence Nightingale Committee.

KEMP, N. 1984. A Place for Quality. *Senior Nurse*, **1**, 34, November 21.

LONG, R. 1981. *Systematic Nursing Care.* London: Faber & Faber.

LUKER, K. A. 1981. An overview of evaluation research in nursing. *Journal of Advanced Nursing*, **6**. 87–93.

LUNT, B. J. & JENKINS, J. 1983. Goal setting in terminal care: a method of recording treatment aims and priorities. *Journal of Advanced Nursing*, **8**. 495–505.

MAYERS, M. G. 1978. *A Systematic Approach to the Nursing Care Plan.* 2nd Ed. New York: Appleton-Century-Crofts.

ROPER, N., LOGAN, W. W. & TIERNEY, A. J. 1980. *The Elements of Nursing.* Edinburgh: Churchill Livingstone.

ROPER, N., LOGAN, W. W. & TIERNEY, A. J. 1983. *Learning to Use the Process of Nursing.* Edinburgh: Churchill Livingstone.

ROPER, N., LOGAN, W. W. & TIERNEY, A. J. 1983. *Models of Nursing.* Edinburgh: Churchill Livingstone.

ROYAL COLLEGE OF NURSING. 1980. *Standards of Nursing Care.* London: Royal College of Nursing.

ROYAL COLLEGE OF NURSING. 1981. *Towards Standards*. London: Royal College of Nursing.

ROYAL COLLEGE OF NURSING. 1986. *Nursing Process*. Report of a Working Party of the RCN Association of Nursing Practice. London: Royal College of Nursing.

STANLEY, B. 1984. Evaluation of treatment goals; the use of goal attainment scaling. *Journal of Advanced Nursing*, **9**. 351–6.

SHEARER, M. S. & SHEARER, D. E. 1972. The Pontage Project – a model for early childhood education. *Exceptional Children*, **38**. 210–17.

WILSON BARNETT, H. J. 1981. Sizing up the scores. A care evaluation feature. *Nursing Mirror*, 26 August. 31–33.

Index

Notes